Made in United States
Orlando, FL
31 May 2022

18363679R00057